THE
40 MOST BEAUTIFUL
Baby Animals
IN THE WORLD

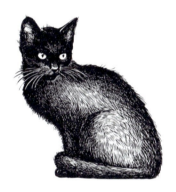

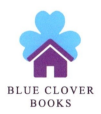

BLUE CLOVER
BOOKS

Copyright © 2022 Blue Clover Books
All Rights Reserved.

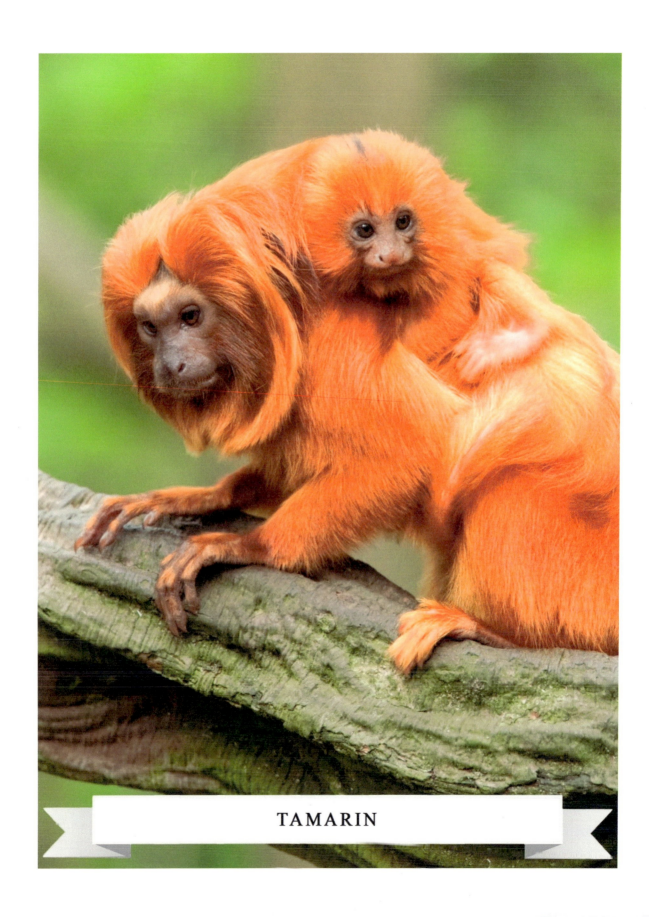

TAMARIN

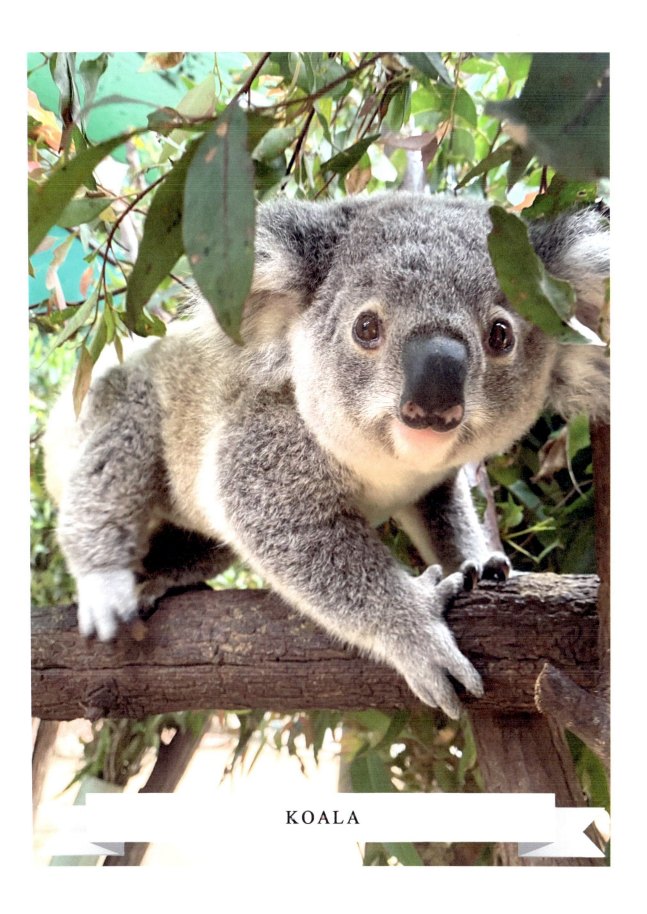
KOALA

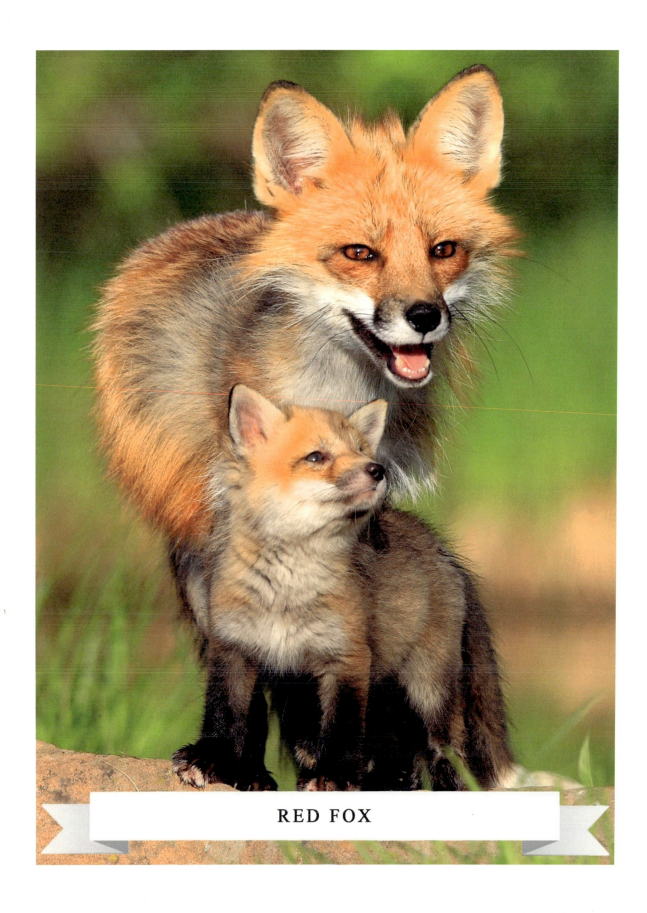

RED FOX

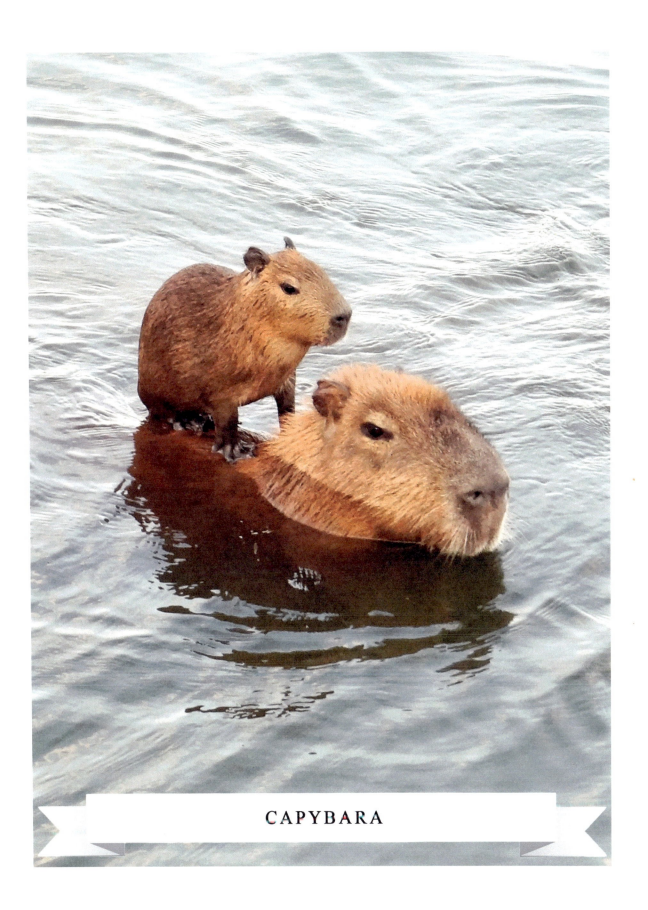

CAPYBARA

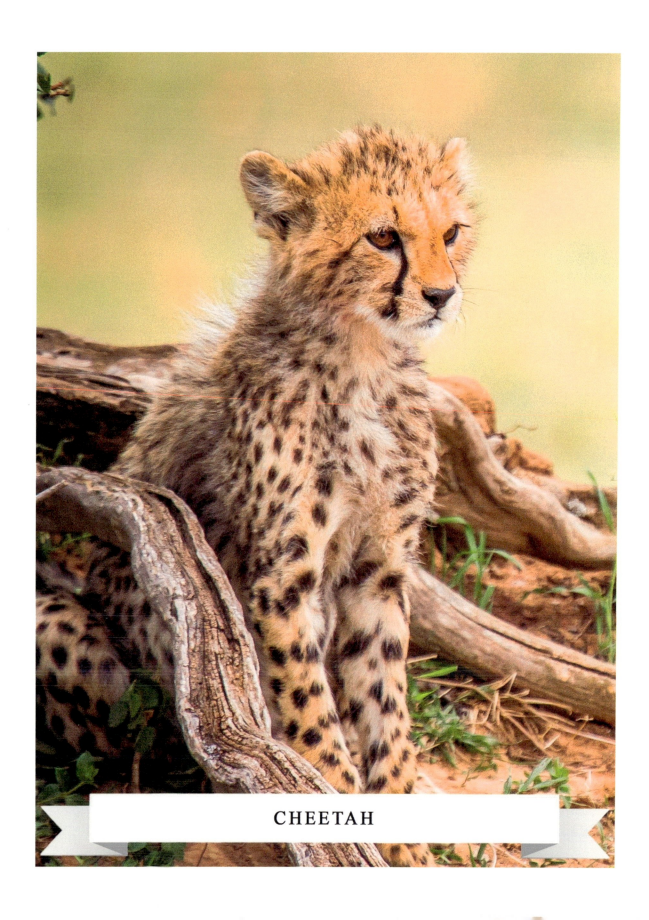

CHEETAH

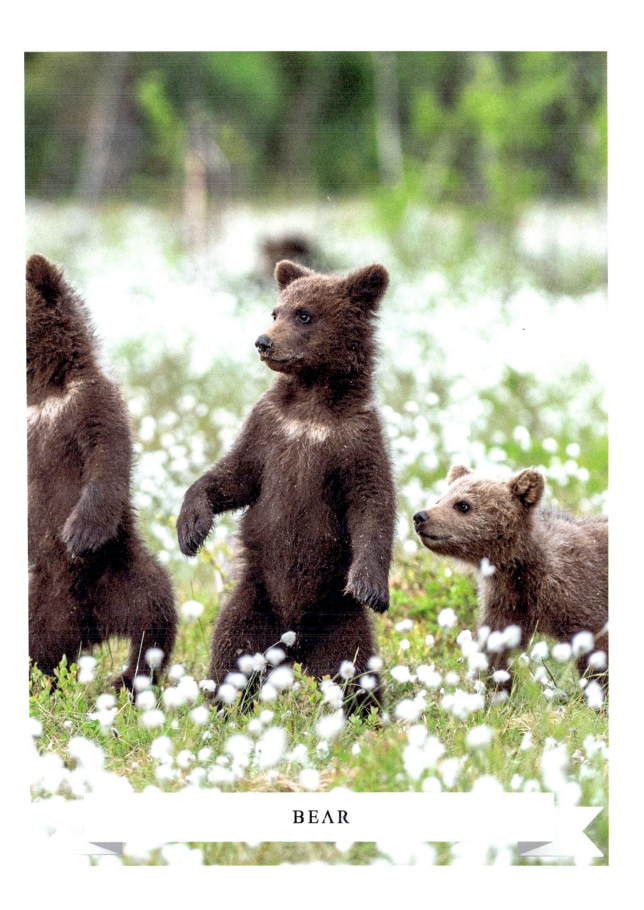

BEAR

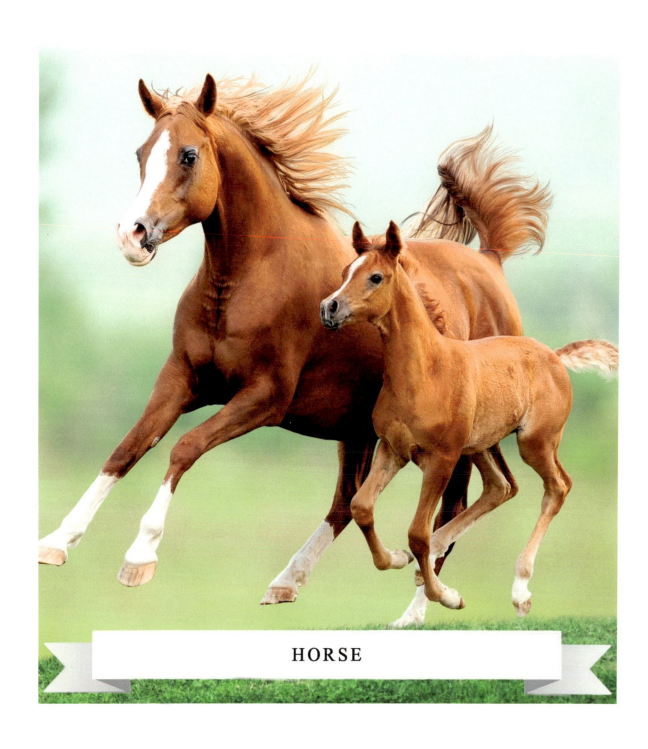

HORSE

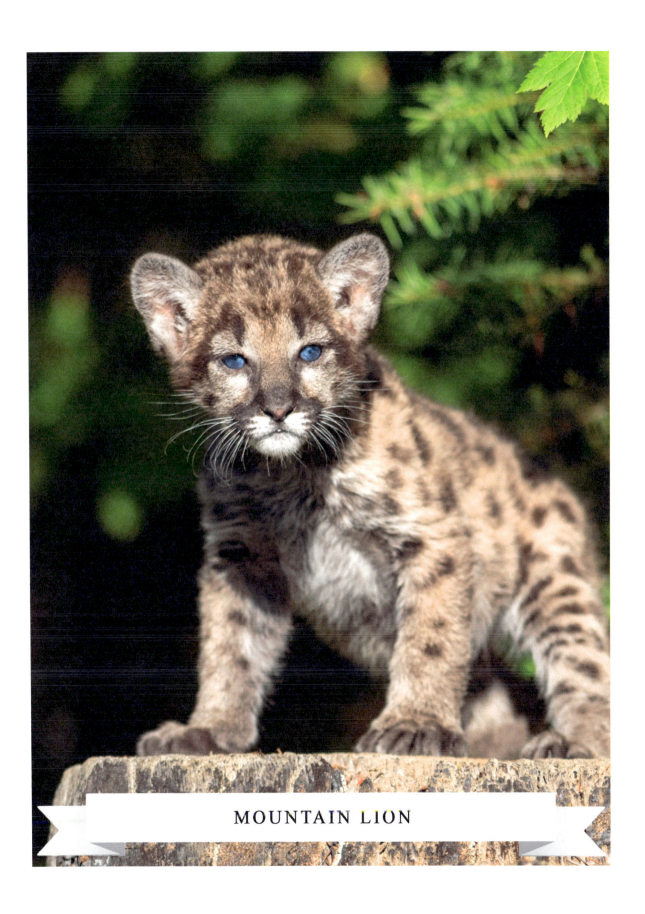

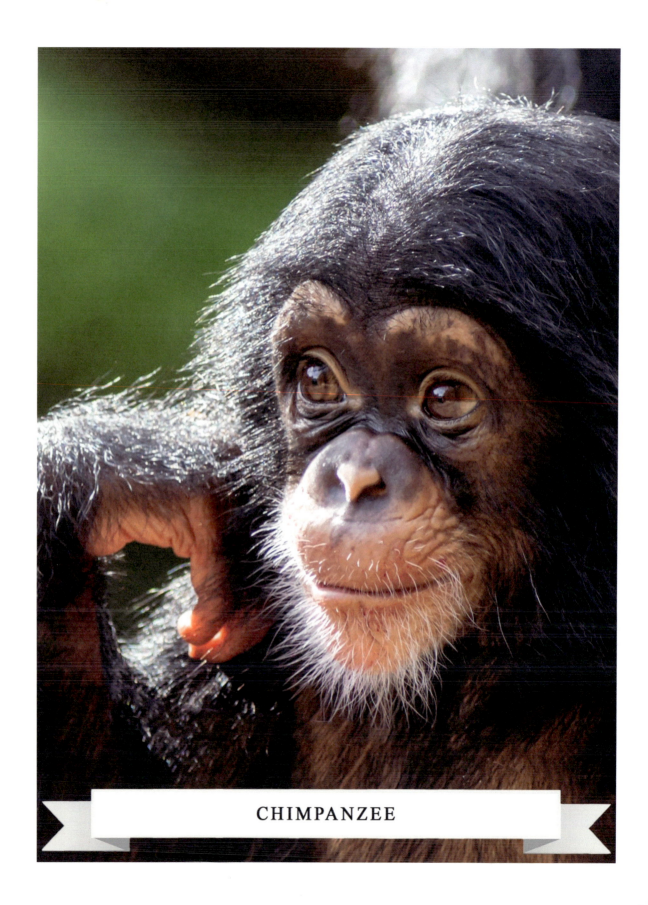
CHIMPANZEE

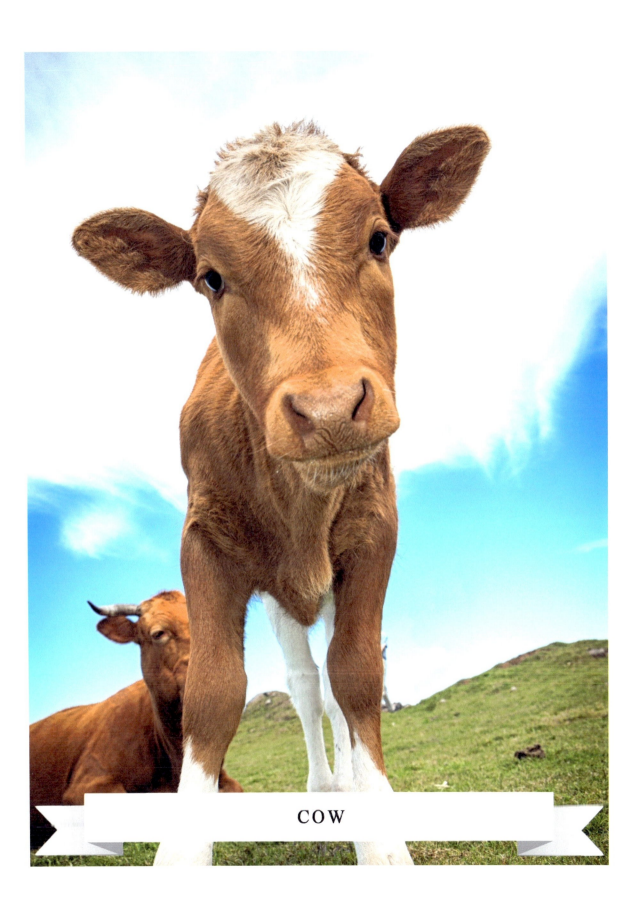

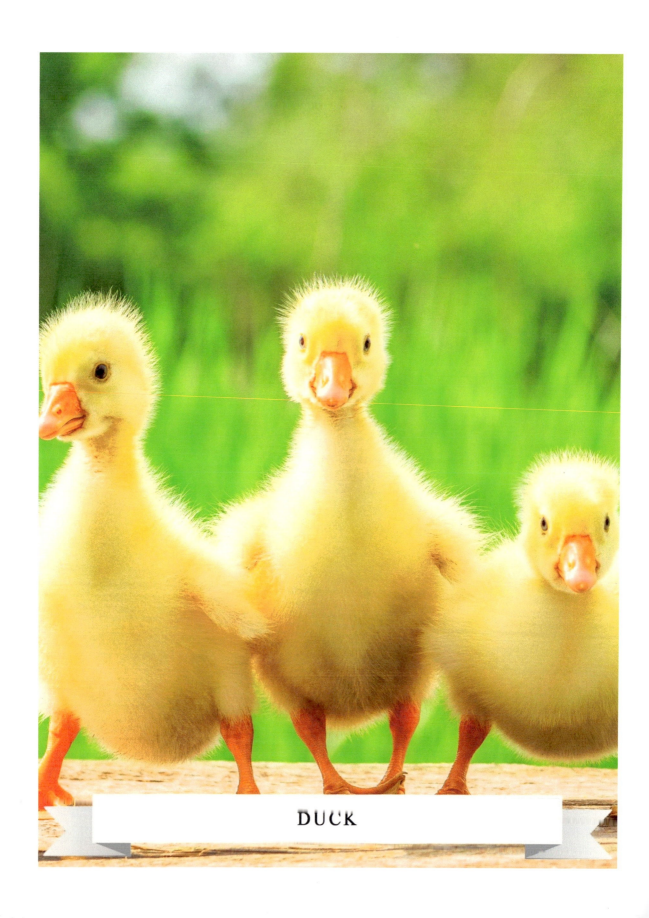

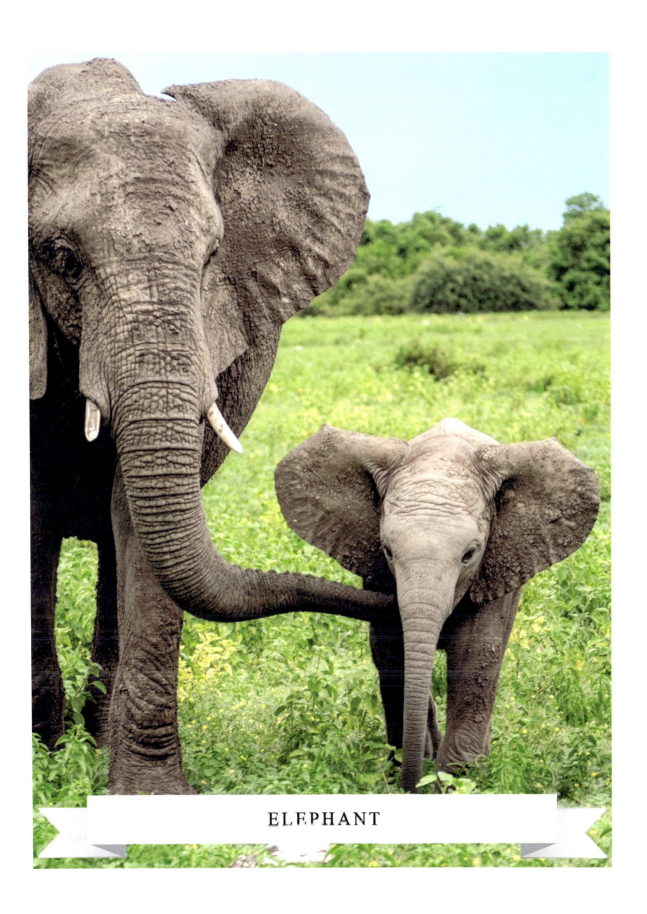
ELEPHANT

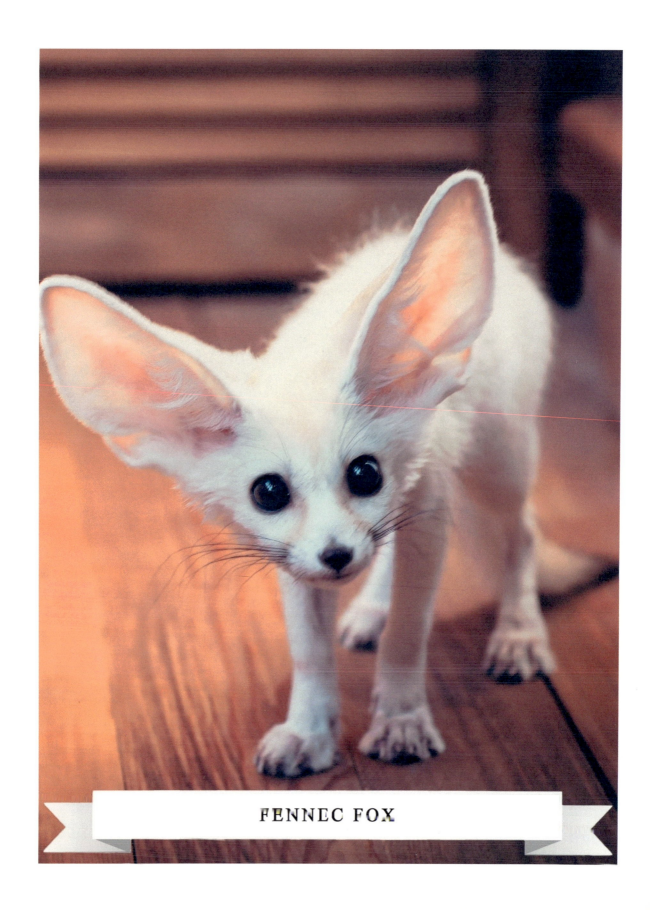
FENNEC FOX

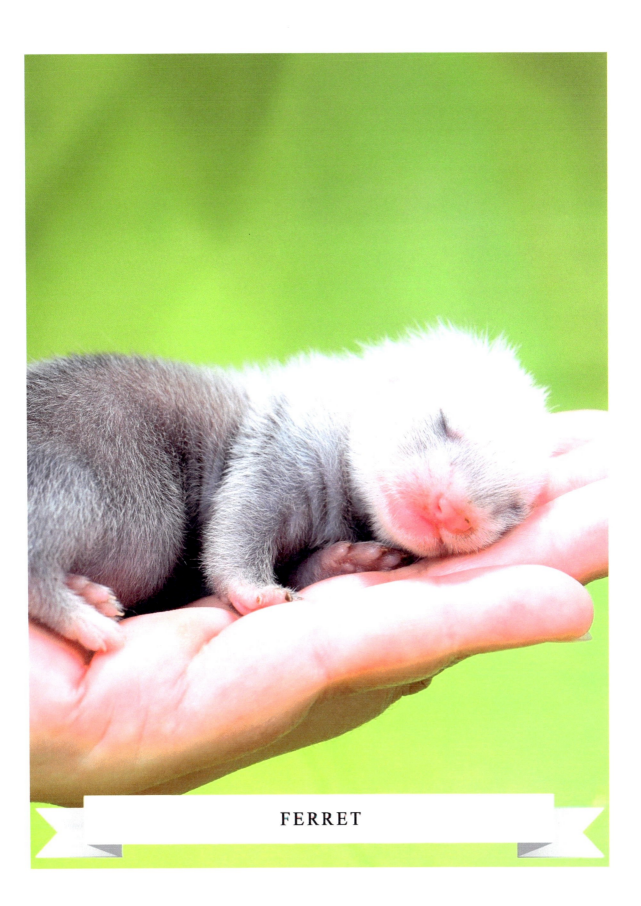

FERRET

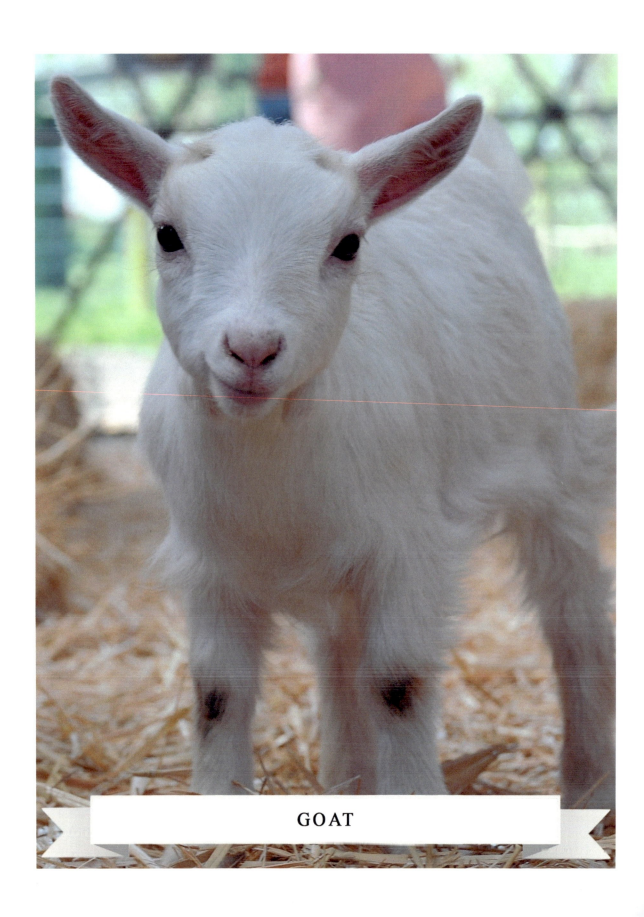

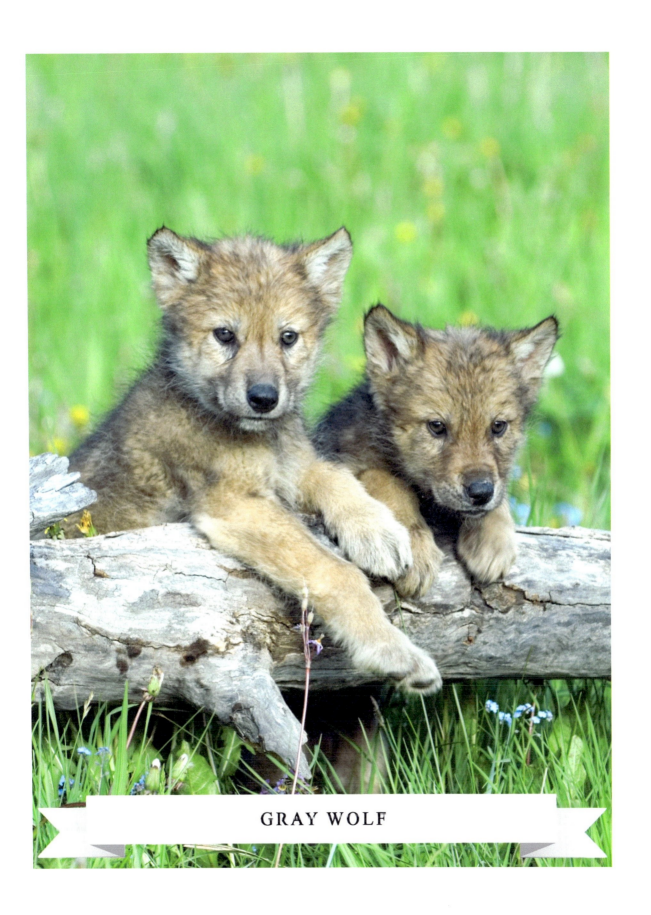
GRAY WOLF

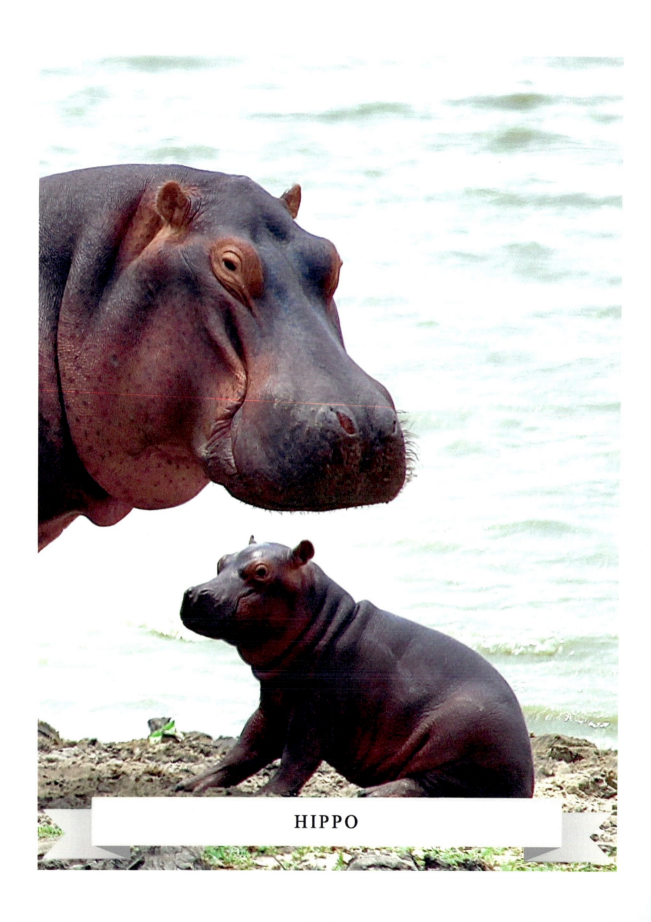

HIPPO

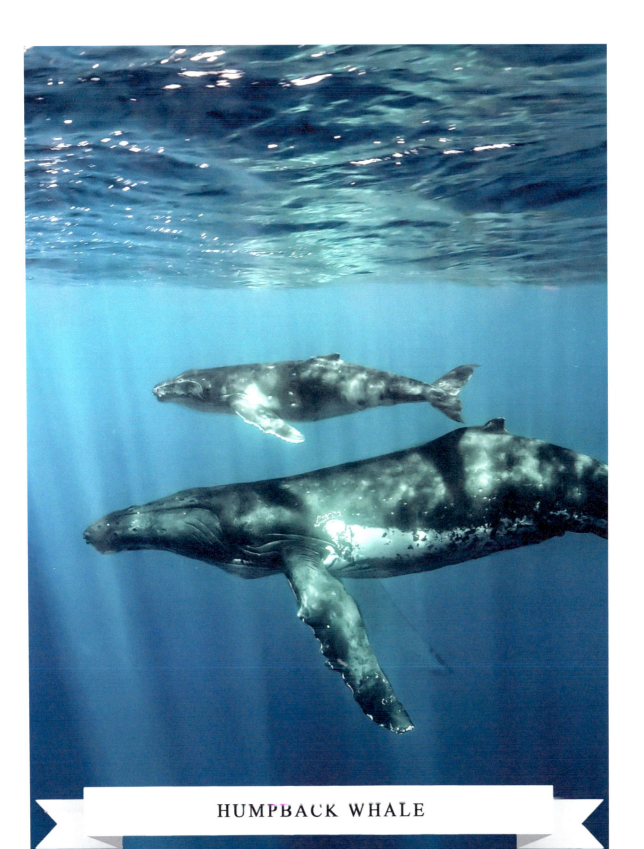

HUMPBACK WHALE

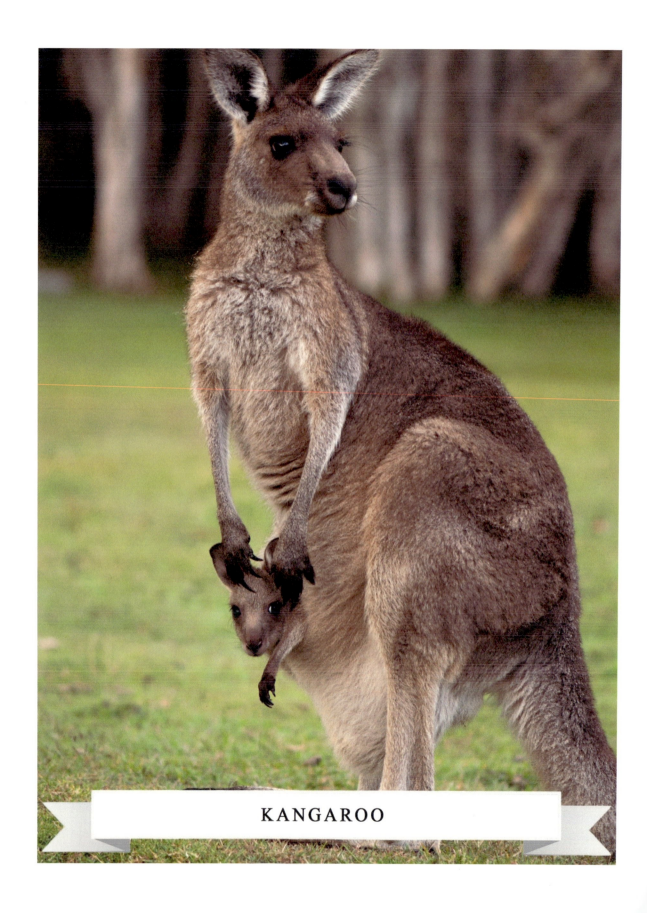

KANGAROO

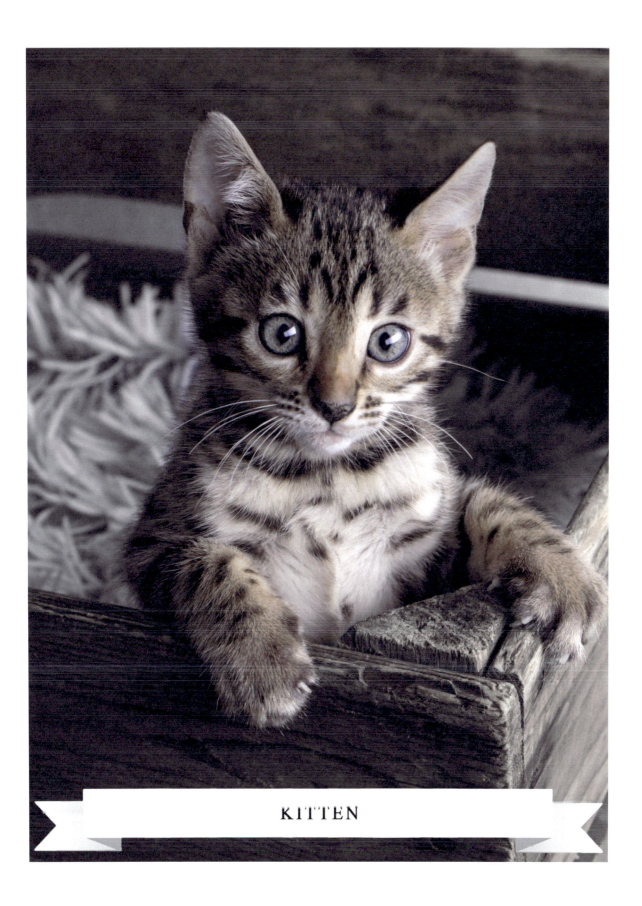

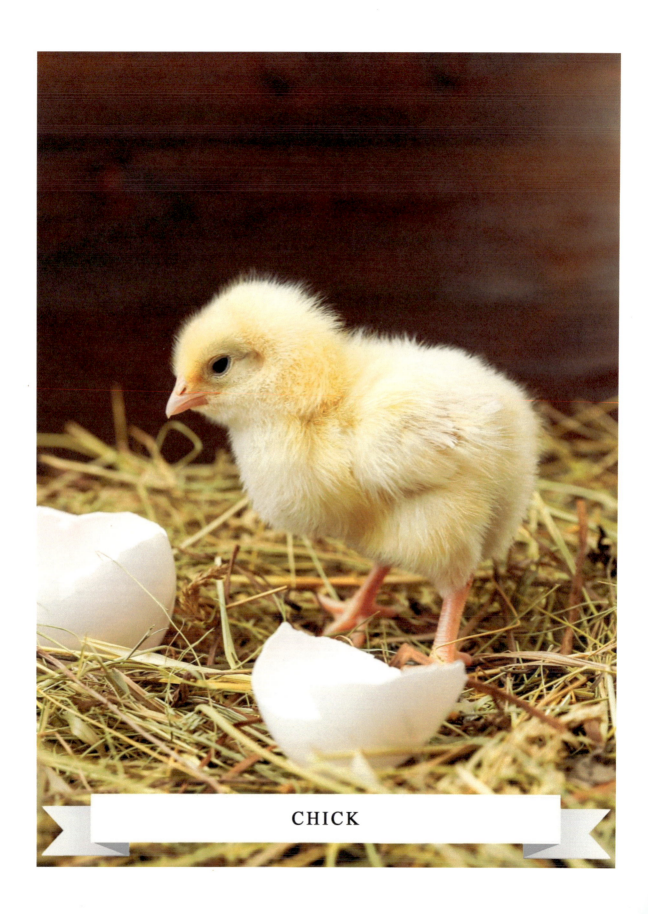

CHICK

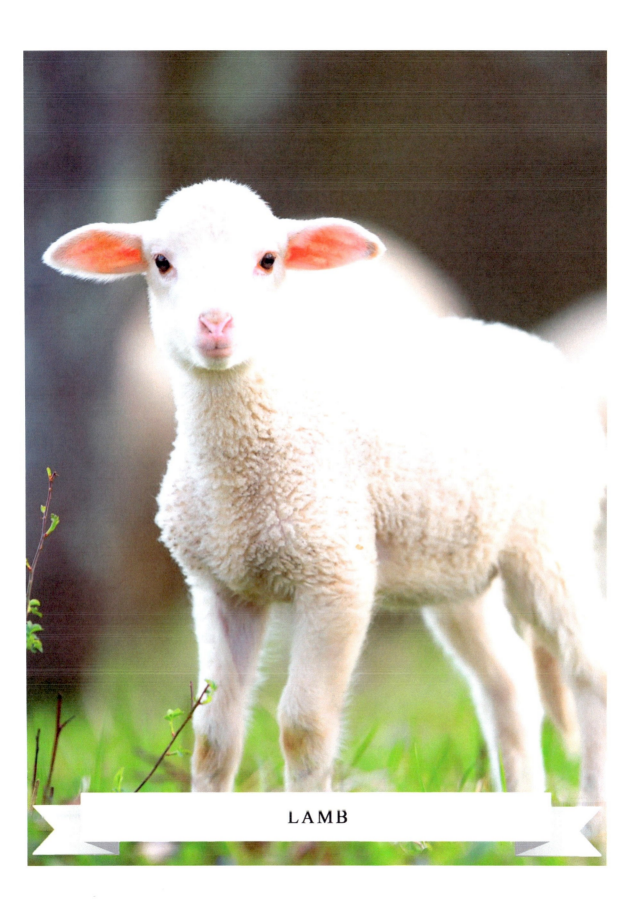

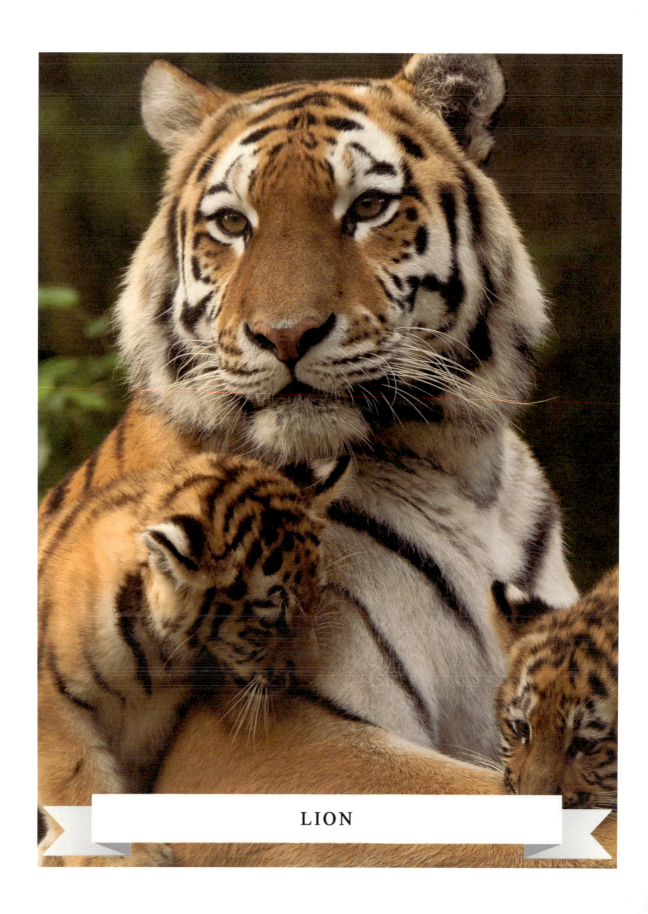

LION

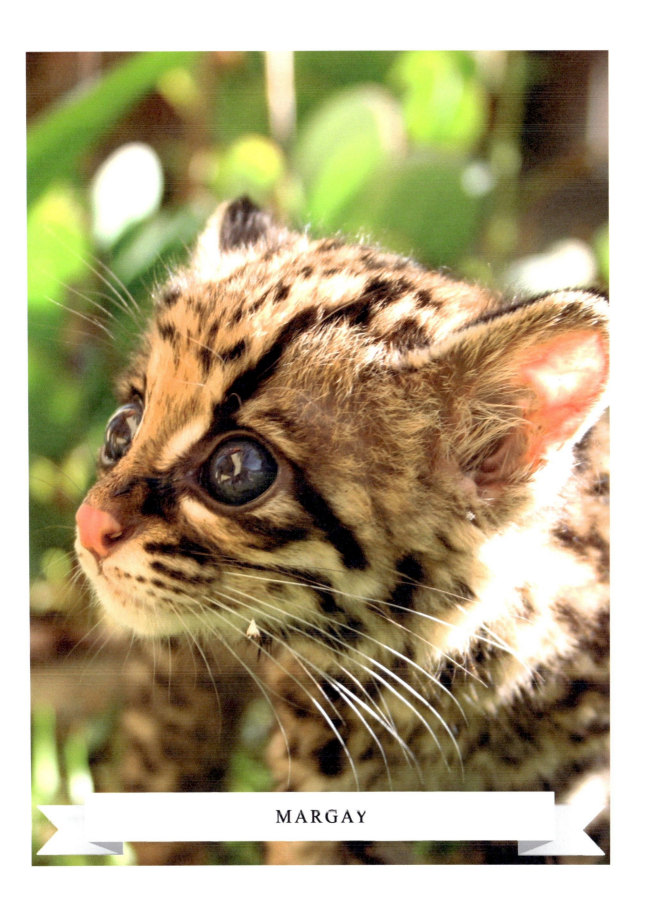

MARGAY

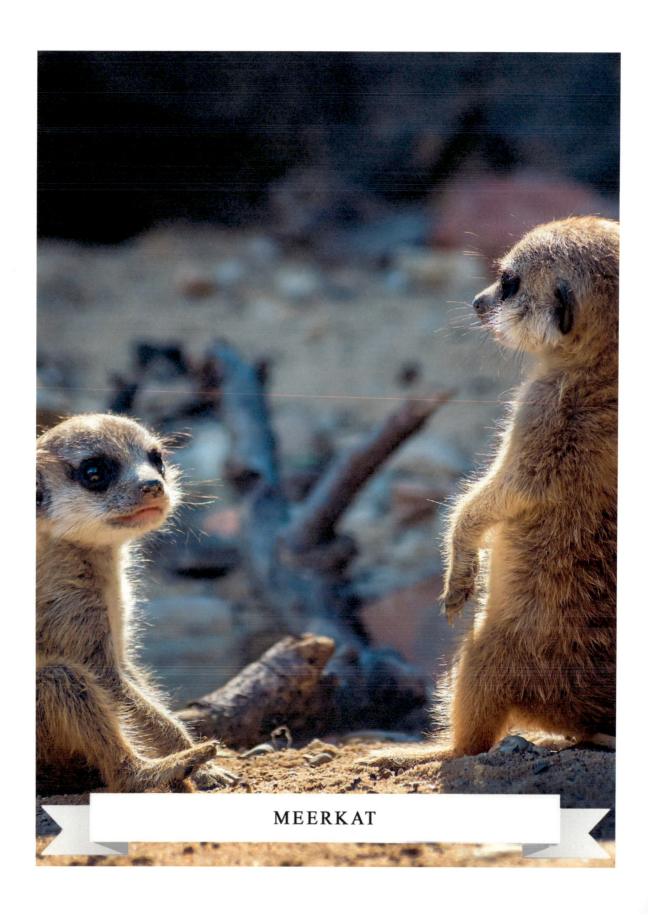

MEERKAT

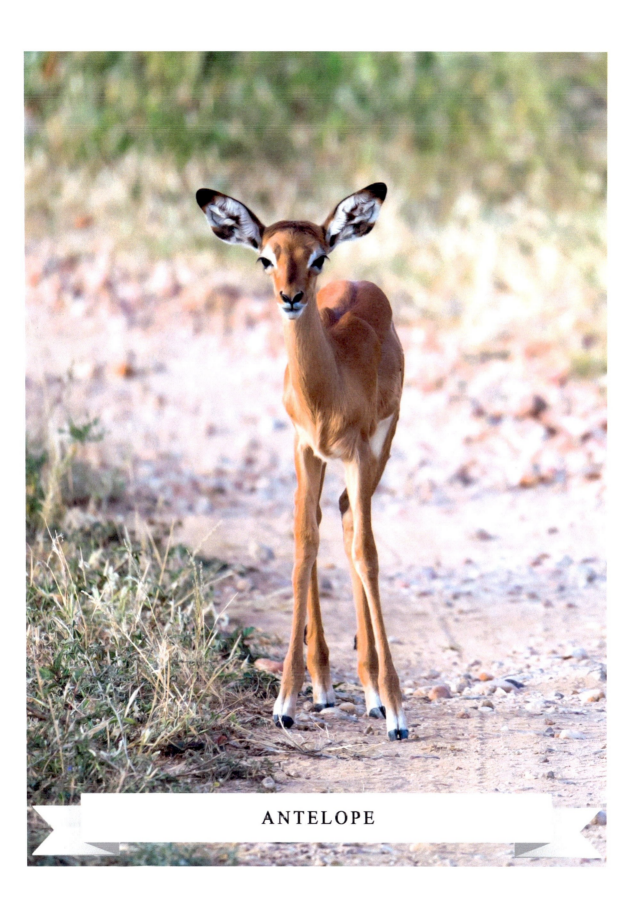
ANTELOPE

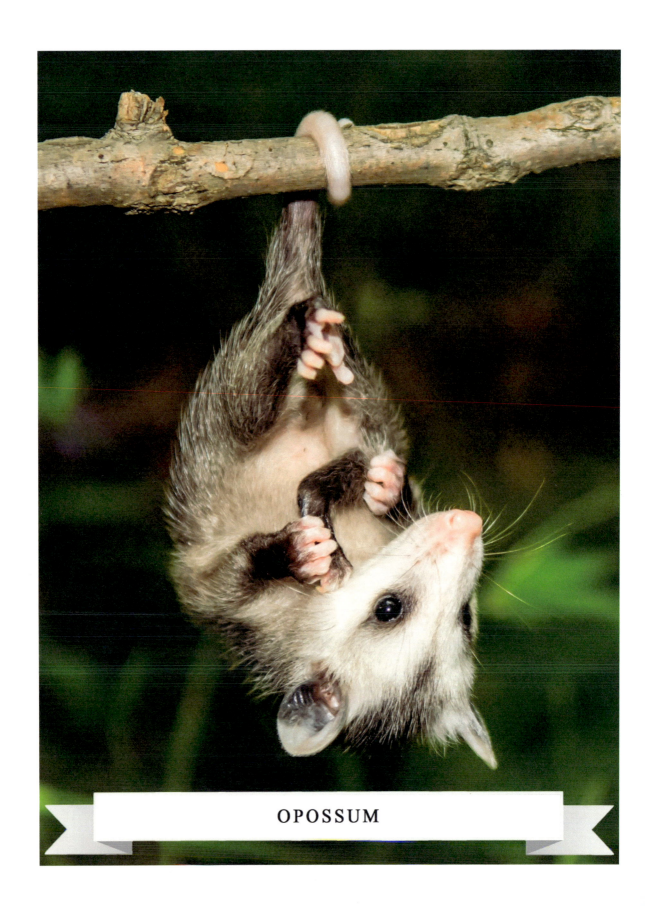

OPOSSUM

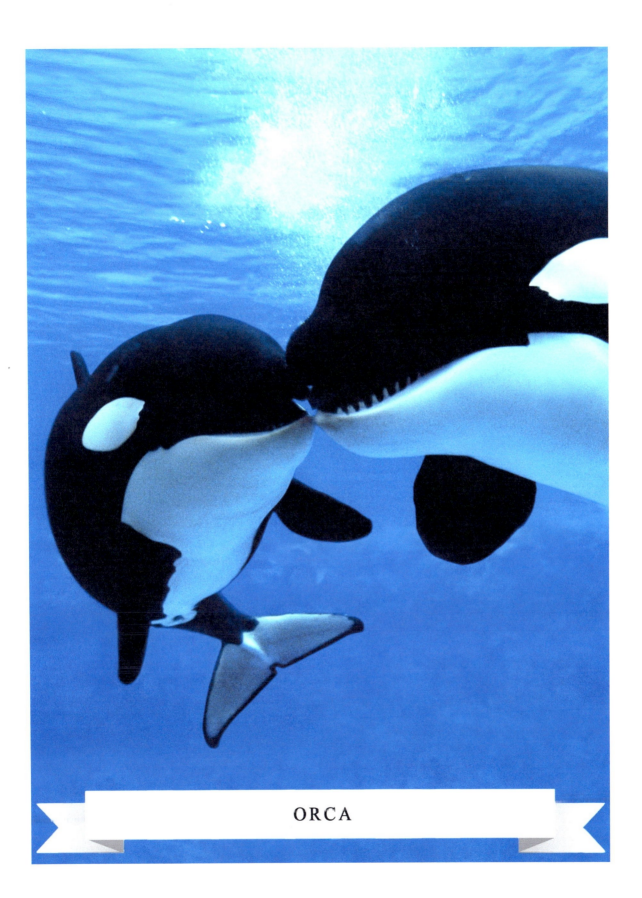

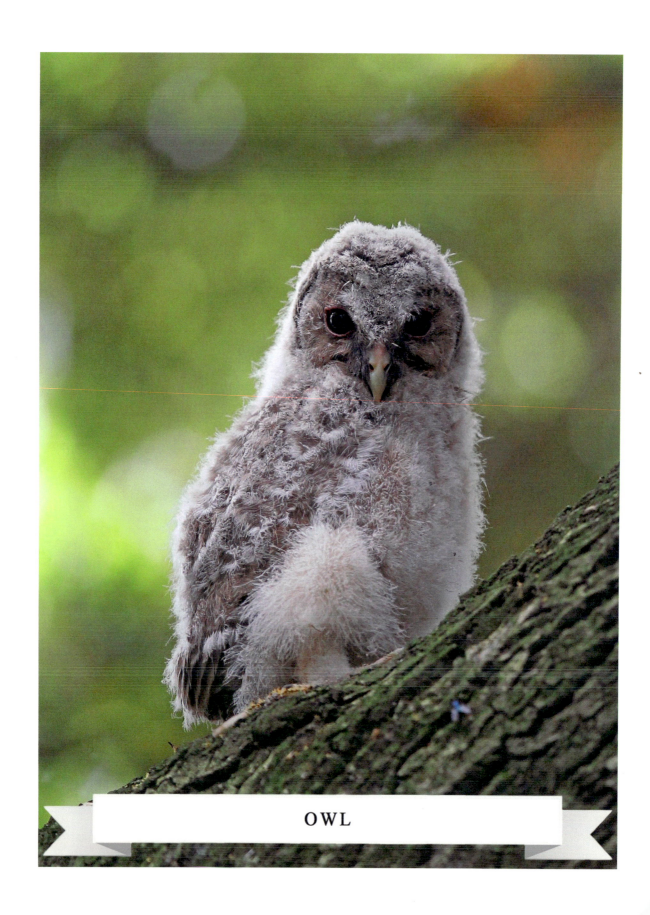

OWL

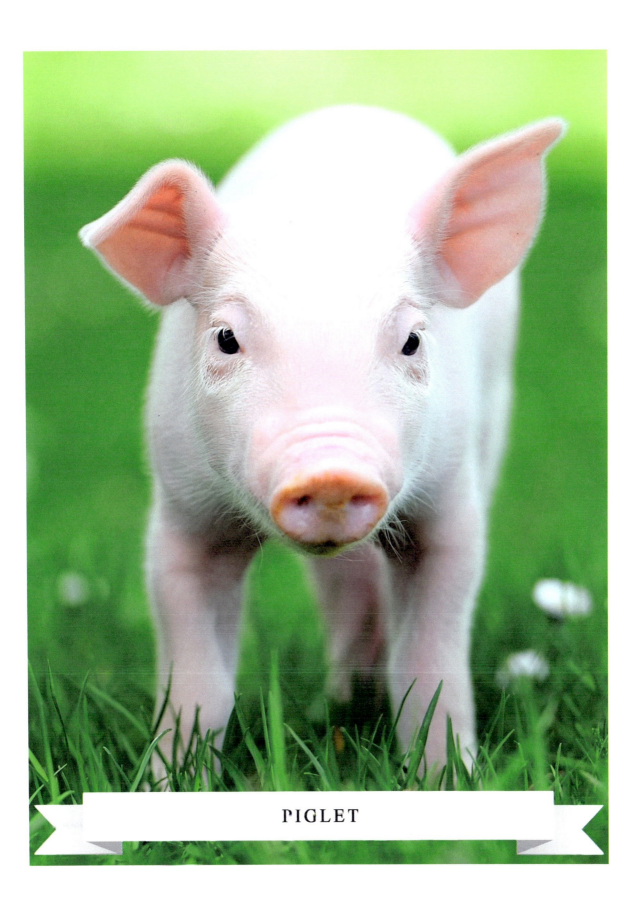

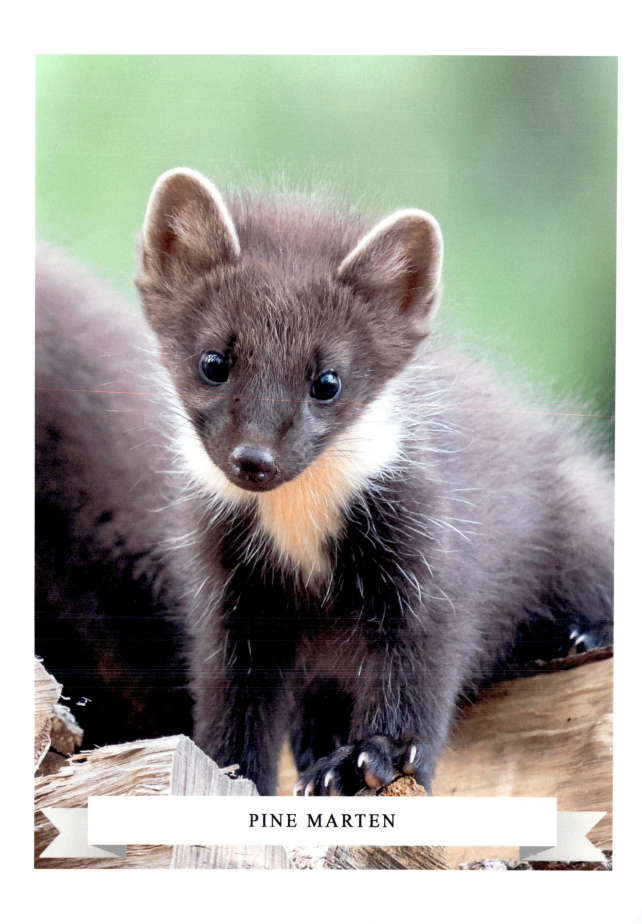

PINE MARTEN

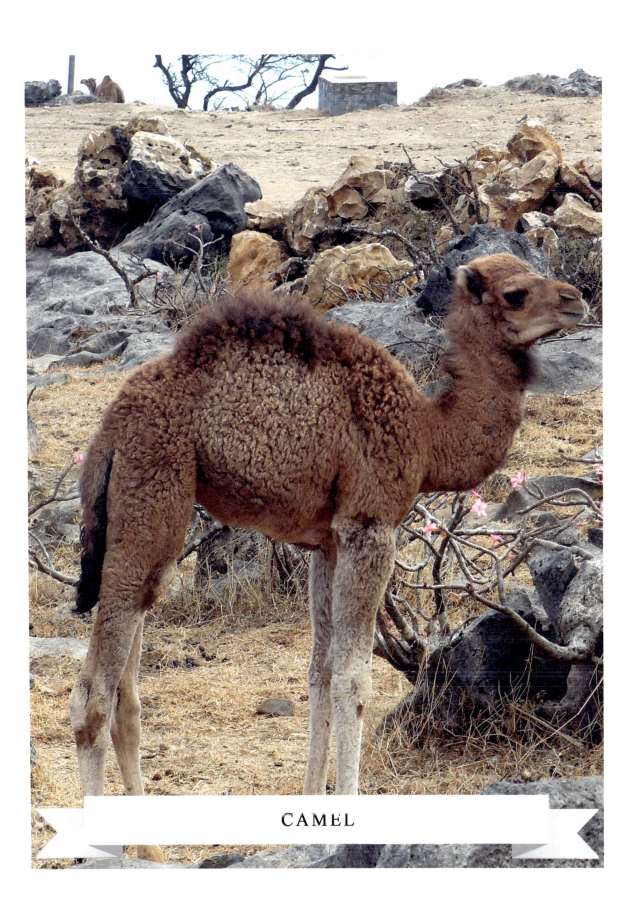
CAMEL

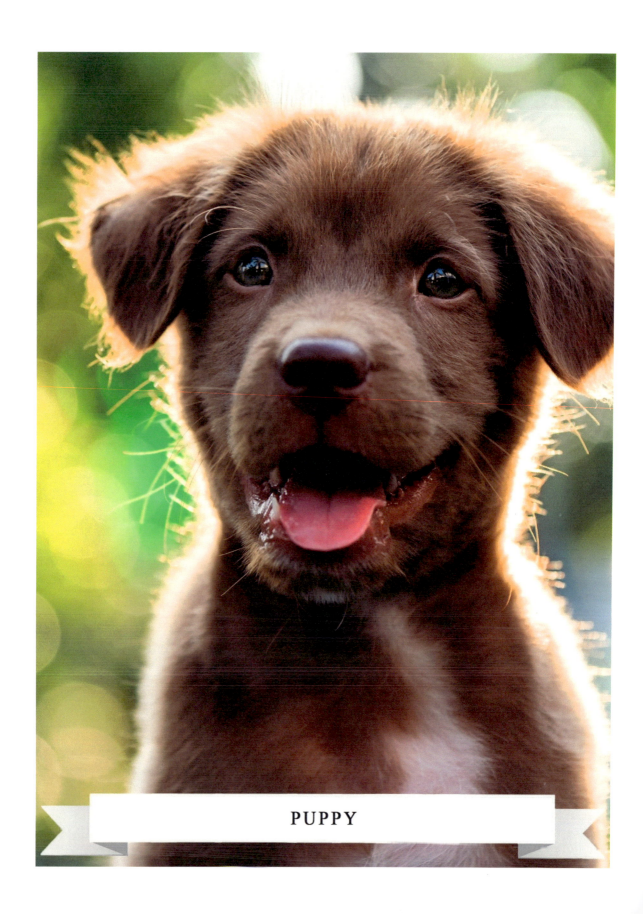
PUPPY

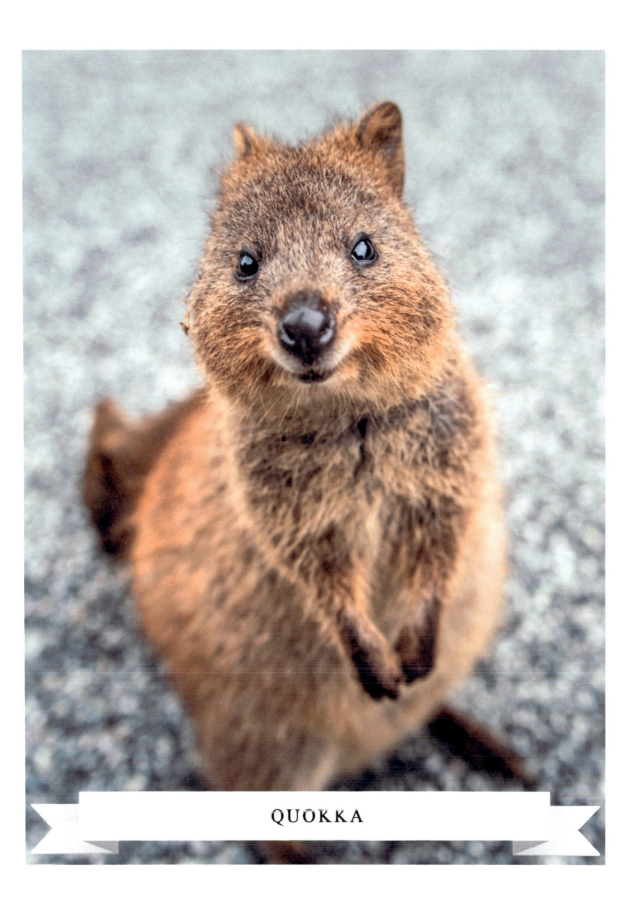

QUOKKA

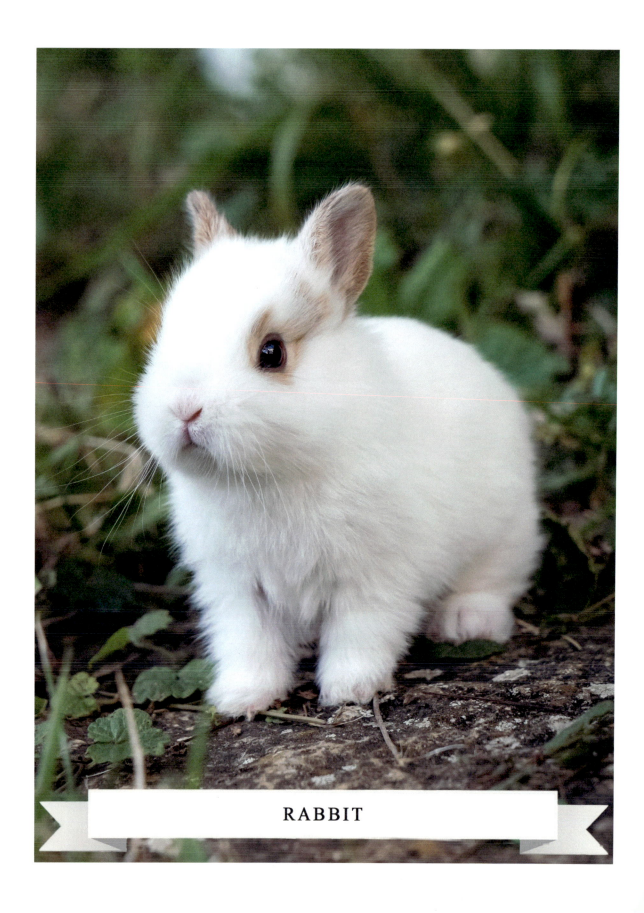

RABBIT

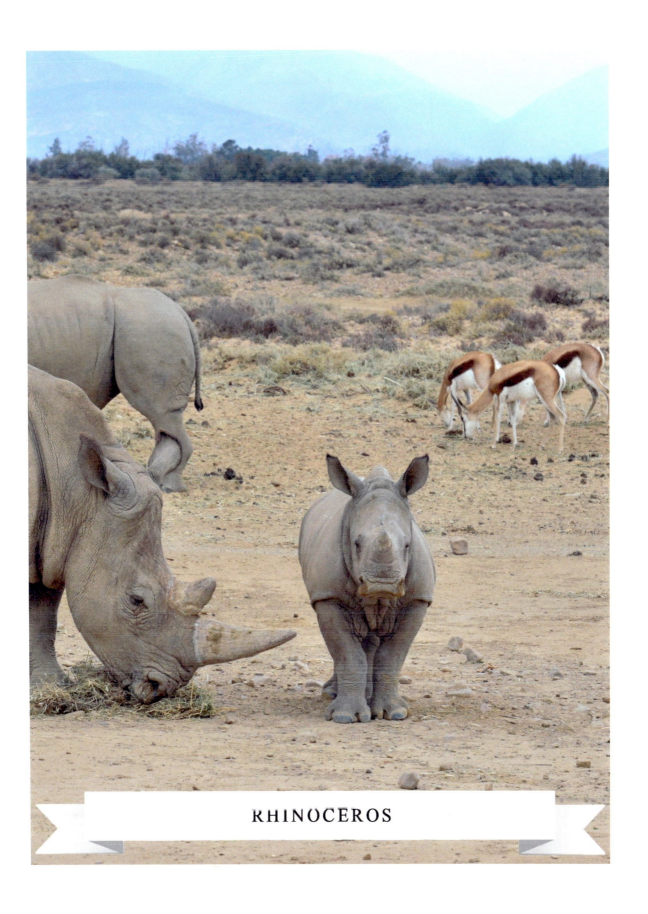

RHINOCEROS

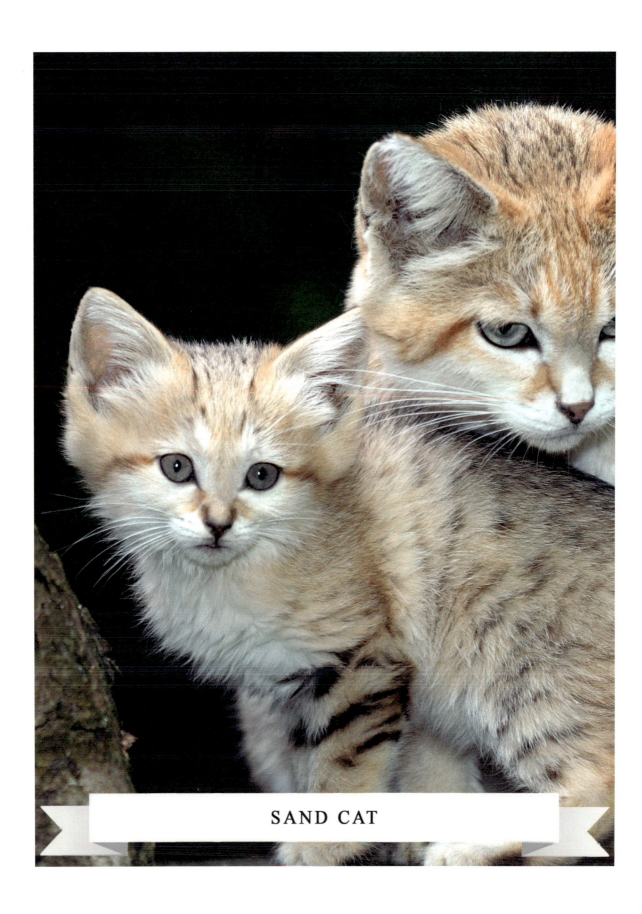

SAND CAT

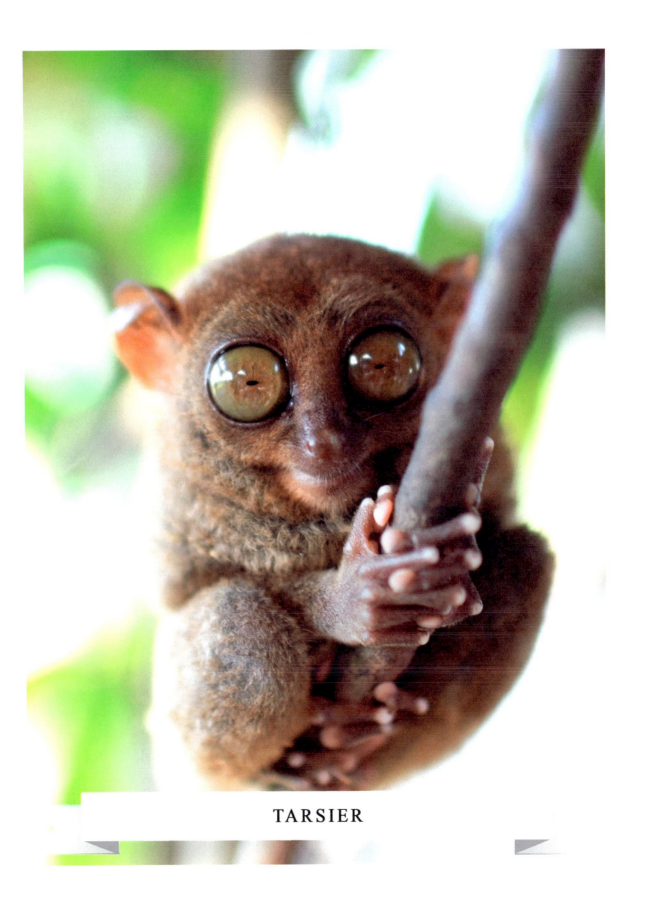

TARSIER

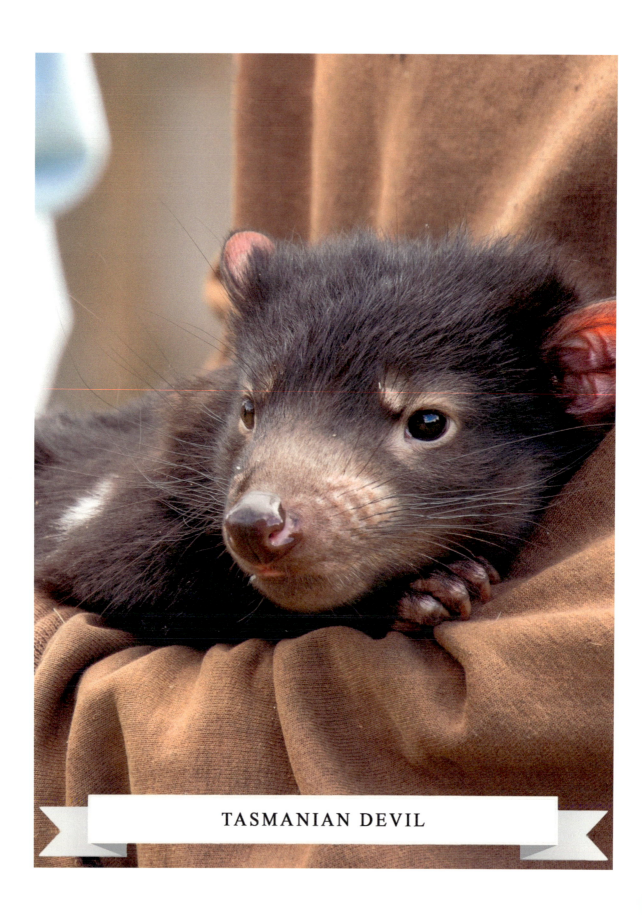

TASMANIAN DEVIL

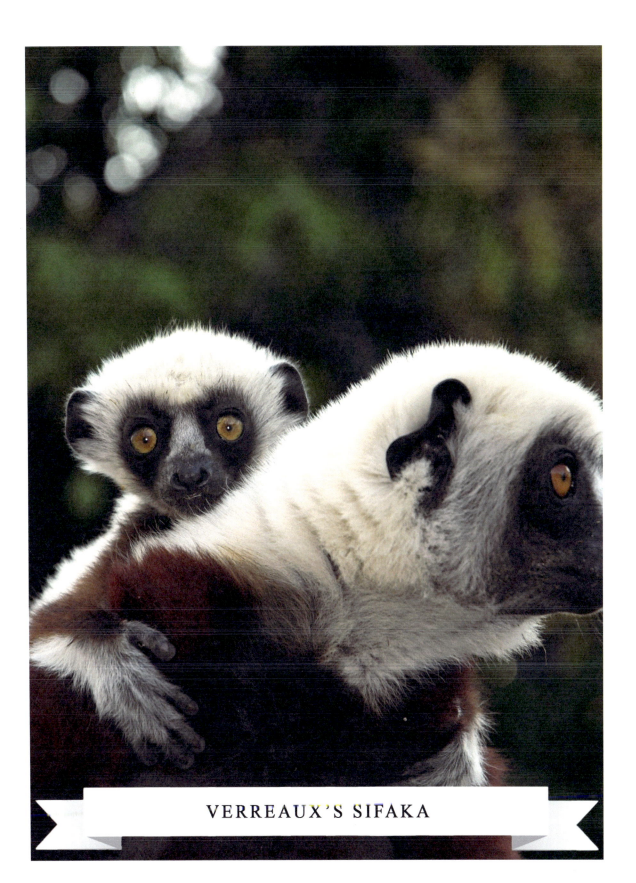
VERREAUX'S SIFAKA

Thank you

Thanks for your interest in our books.

Please consider purchasing our other books available now at Amazon.com.

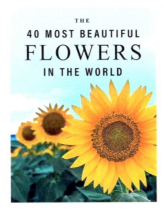
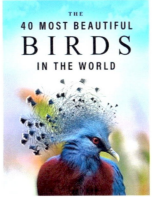
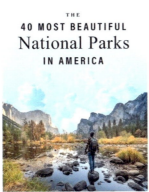
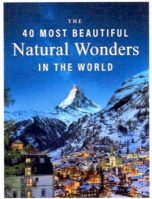

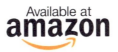

(Just search for "Blue Clover Books" on Amazon.)

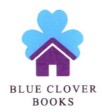

Made in the USA
Columbia, SC
08 June 2024

36848659R00024